Published By Nicholas Thompson

@ Irvin Denis

Pizza: A Wide Variety of Pizza Recipes and Good Tasty Pizza

All Right RESERVED

ISBN 978-1-7782903-1-2

TABLE OF CONTENTS

the Best Basis For Pizza 1

The Dough For Pies, Pies And Pizzas 3

Pizza Grilled Peach Pizza 5

Pizza Breakfast Pizza 10

Apple And Bacon Pita Pizzas Recipe 13

Bacon Pickle Pizza 15

Zucchini Soup 17

Cucumber Soup 19

Pizza With Potatoes And Mozzarella 20

Pizza With Onion And Asparagus 22

Crispy Crust Dough 24

No-Rise Pizza Dough 26

Fast Pizza For Baking 27

Quick Pizza Dough 29

Pizza Fruit Pizza 31

Pizza Stuff Crust Chipotle Chicken Pizza 34

Bacon Weave Pizza 38

Ban Mi Pizza	40
Vegetarian Minestrone Soup	43
Cabbage Stew	45
Pizza With Prosciutto And Tomatoes	47
Pizza With Cheese And Pesto	49
Spicy Pizza With Sausages	51
Mama's Best Crust	54
Honey And Whole Wheat Dough	56
Pizza Dough In The Bread Maker	58
Pizza Minute	60
Home Fast Pizza	63
Pizza Roasted Garlic And Mushroom Pizza	65
Pizza Grilled Prosciutto, Spinach, And Burrito Pizza	68
Pizza Grilled Strawberry Balsamic Herb Pizza	71
Bbq Chicken Crust Pizza	74
Bbq Chicken Pizza	76
Bbq Chicken Pizza Sliders	78
Chicken Rice Soup	80

- Miso Soup 82
- Grilled Pizza From Mario Batali 84
- Pizza Bbq Chicken 87
- Pizza With Grilled Vegetables 90
- Master Pizza Dough 92
- Rye Dough 94
- Pizza With Sausage 96
- The Dough For Pizza Without Yeast 99
- Pizza Low Carb Crust Less Pizza 100
- Pizza Grilled Home Style Pizza With Honey Sriracha Glaze 101
- Bbq Chicken Skillet Pizza 104
- Bbq Pizza With Slaw Recipe 106
- Grilled Pizza 110
- Pizza Margarita With Two Grilled Cheeses 113
- Grilled Avocado With Tomato Salsa 116
- Deep Dish Pizza Dough 118
- Basic Pizza Sauce 120

Heirloom Pizza Sauce	122
Pizza Tentazione	124
Pizza Dough With Cheese	128
Pizza Roasted Garlic Lasagna Pizza	130
Pizza Blt Ranch Flatbread Pizza	134
Fast On Bread Pizza	136
Pizza With Salami And Tomato	138
Pizza Turkey Pizza	140
Captain America Pizza	142
Carne Asada Pizza Recipe	144
Cauliflower Breakfast Pizza	148
Individual Pizza Doughs	151

The Best Basis For Pizza

Ingredients:

- 1 1/2 cup (350 ml), warm water (45 C)
- 1 tsp salt
- 2 tbsp. olive oil
- 3 1/3 cups (425 g) flour
- 2 1/4 tsp (7 g), active dry yeast
- 1/2 tsp Sahara

Directions:
1. In a large bowl, dissolve yeast and sugar in warm water, let stand 10 minutes.
2. In the yeast mixture, add salt and oil. Stir in half of the flour.
3. Turn dough out onto a clean, heavily floured surface and add more flour.
4. Knead until the dough will not cease to be sticky.

5. Place the dough in a bowl greased with stretching.
6. Butter and cover with a damp cloth. Let the dough rise until it will increase in volume by half, about 1 hour.
7. Crumple the dough and form a tight ball.
8. Allow the dough to rest a moment before rolling.
9. Roll out and add your sauce and toppings.
10. Preheat oven to 220 C. If you bake the dough on a pizza stone, then lay the filling on the dough and bake immediately.
11. If you bake a pizza on a baking sheet, then lightly grease it with oil and let the dough rise 15 20 minutes before adding the filling and baking.
12. Bake the pizza in the preheated oven, until cheese and crust are golden, 15 to 20 minutes.

The Dough For Pies, Pies And Pizzas

Ingredients:

- 200 g butter or margarine
- 1 egg
- 1/2 tsp salt
- 3 cups flour (400 g)
- 7 g (2.5 teaspoons) active dry yeast or 25 g fresh
- 3/4 cup milk
- 2 tsp granulated sugar

Directions:

1. Yeast breed in warm milk 2 tsp Sahara. Let stand 10 minutes, until the foam.
2. Melt the butter or margarine, cool slightly. In a large bowl, beat the egg with salt, add the yeast to the milk and melted butter.
3. Add the flour, knead the dough. The dough should be soft, come off the hands, not steep.

4. You can cook immediately or refrigerate for several hours or even days.
5. Roll out, sprinkle with flour if sticky.
6. Bake at 190° C until golden brown.

Pizza Grilled Peach Pizza

Ingredients:

Pizza dough

- 1 1/2 teaspoons salt
- Jalapeño Honey
- ½ cup honey
- 1-2 jalapenos, sliced
- 1/2 cup warm water
- 1 1/2 teaspoons active dry yeast
- 1 1/2 cups flour

Pizza

- 4 ounces mozzarella cheese, shredded
- 4 ounces gorgonzola cheese, crumbled
- 8 slices thick cut bacon, fried
- 1 tablespoon olive oil
- 2 peaches, sliced into wedges

- ½ cup basil pesto
- 1 cup cherry tomatoes, halved
- 2 cups butter lettuce, baby kale or arugula

Directions:

Pizza dough

1. In a large bowl, combine water and yeast. Mix with a spoon, then let sit until foamy, about 5 minutes. Add in the flour and salt, stirring with a spoon until the dough comes together but is still sticky.
2. Using your hands, on a floured surface, form the dough into a ball and if needed, work the additional 1/2-cup flour into the dough. All of the mixing and kneading can also be done in a stand mixer with the dough hook attachment.
3. Next, rub the same bowl with olive oil, then place the dough inside, turning to coat.
4. Cover with a towel and place in a warm area while you prepare the pesto; let sit at least 20 minutes.

Jalapeño honey

1. In a small saucepan bring the honey to a low boil.
2. Add the jalapeños and cook one minute longer. Remove from the heat.
3. Store in an airtight container in the fridge for up to one week. Warm again before serving.

Pizza

1. Heat a grill or grill pan to high heat. Toss the peaches with the olive oil. Once the grill is hot, place the peaches on the grill and grill until char marks appear, about 2 minutes per side. Remove from the grill and set aside.
2. Preheat you Cuisinart Outdoor Pizza Oven to 500 degrees F.
3. Lightly flour a counter. Use your hands or a rolling pin to roll the pizza dough out until you have a flattened disk.
4. Then use your hands to gently tug, pull and push the pizza dough into a rough 10-12 inch

circle. Dust your pizza peel with a generous amount of flour.
5. Spread the pesto all over the pizza crust.
6. Top with mozzarella and crumbled gorgonzola. Sprinkle the bacon over top and then arrange the peaches over the cheese.*
7. Once your pizza oven is preheated, carefully slide your pizza from the peel and onto the pizza stone.
8. Bake for 8-10 minutes or until the cheese is melted and bubbly. To remove the pizza, slide the peel under the pizza and pull the pizza out.
9. Top the pizza with cherry tomatoes, basil and lettuce.
10. Drizzle with jalapeno honey and EAT!
11. If you prefer, you can add the grilled peaches after the pizza is done cooking. However, I think I liked the pizza best when the peaches were cooked onto the pizza.

12. If you do not have a pizza oven, you can bake the pizza at 425 degrees for 15 to 20 minutes OR if using a pizza stone, 500 degrees F. for 10 minutes.

Pizza Breakfast Pizza

Ingredients:

- 2 ounces (1/2 cup) shredded mozzarella cheese
- 8 cherry tomatoes, sliced
- 4 large eggs
- 2 strips cooked center cut bacon, chopped
- 1 cup (5 oz) all purpose or white whole wheat flour*
- 1 1/2 teaspoons baking powder
- 1/2 teaspoon kosher salt
- 1 cup non-fat greek yogurt (not regular), drained if theres any liquid
- Handful baby spinach

Directions:

1. Preheat the oven to 450F. Place a silicone liner on a large baking sheet or spray with oil if using parchment.
2. In a medium bowl combine the flour, baking powder and salt and whisk well.
3. Add the yogurt and mix with a fork or spatula until well combined, it will look like small crumbles.
4. Lightly dust flour on a work surface and remove dough from the bowl, knead the dough a few times until dough is tacky, but not sticky, about 20 turns (it should not leave dough on your hand when you pull away).
5. Divide into 4 equal balls about 3-3/8 oz each.
6. Sprinkle a work surface and rolling pin with a little flour roll the dough out into thin ovals 7 to 8 inches in diameter and place on the prepared baking sheet.

7. Top with spinach, mozzarella and tomatoes, leaving the center open for the egg. Gently break an egg the center of each dough and finish with bacon.
8. Bake 10 to 12 minutes, until the crust is golden and the egg is set. Season with salt and pepper.

Apple And Bacon Pita Pizzas Recipe

Ingredients:

- 4 (6-inch) whole-wheat pitas
- 2 teaspoons olive oil
- 2 ounces cheddar cheese, shredded (about 1/2 cup)
- 2 cups thinly sliced Fuji apple 3 tablespoons grated fresh Parmesan cheese
- 2 tablespoons chopped walnuts toasted
- 1 teaspoon chopped fresh thyme
- 2 apple wood-smoked bacon slices, chopped and cooked

Directions:
1. Preheat broiler to high.
2. Broil pitas 1 minute or until lightly golden.
3. Remove from oven; carefully flip pitas over.

4. Brush evenly with essential olive oil. Sprinkle cheddar over pitas; arrange apple slices over cheese.
5. Sprinkle Parmesan cheese, walnuts, thyme, and bacon evenly over apples.
6. Go back to oven; broil one to two 2 minutes.

Bacon Pickle Pizza

Ingredients:

- 3/4 cup dill pickle slices
- 4 slices bacon , cooked and chopped
- 1 tablespoon freshly chopped dill
- 1/2 teaspoon crushed red pepper flakes
- ranch dressing, for serving, optional
- 2 tablespoons extra-virgin olive oil
- 1 teaspoon garlic powder
- 1 teaspoon italian seasoning
- 1 premade pizza crust
- 1 1/2 cups . mozzarella
- 1/4 cup freshly grated parmesan

Directions:

1. Preheat oven to 375° and line an enormous baking sheet with parchment paper.

2. In a medium bowl, whisk together oil, garlic powder, and Italian seasoning.
3. Place pizza crust on prepared baking sheet and brush around with oil mixture.
4. Top crust with mozzarella and Parmesan and bake until cheese is melty, quarter-hour.
5. Top with pickles and bacon and bake 5 minutes more.
6. Top with dill and red pepper flakes before serving with ranch, if using.

Zucchini Soup

Ingredients:

- ¼ tsp salt
- ¼ tsp pepper
- 1 can vegetable broth
- 1 cup heavy cream
- 1 tablespoon olive oil
- 1 lb. zucchini
- ¼ red onion
- ½ cup all-purpose flour

Directions:

1. In a saucepan heat olive oil and sauté zucchini until tender
2. Add remaining Ingredients: to the saucepan and bring to a boil
3. When all the vegetables are tender transfer to a blender and blend until smooth

4. Pour soup into bowls, garnish with parsley and serve

Cucumber Soup

Ingredients:

- ¼ cup parsley
- ¼. cup cilantro
- ¼ cup greens
- 1 cup baby spinach
- 2 cups cucumber
- 2 tablespoons olive oil
- 2 cloves garlic
- ¼ cup lemon juice
- Salt
- radishes

Directions:

1. In a blender add all Ingredients: and blend until smooth
2. Season and refrigerate the soup
3. When ready pour soup into bowl and serve

Pizza With Potatoes And Mozzarella

Ingredients:

- Cornmeal 2 tablespoons
- Smoked mozzarella cheese 250 g
- Basil 50g Tomatoes 2 pieces
- Salt to taste
- Ground black pepper to taste
- Wheat flour 300 g
- Olive oil 4 tablespoons
- Dry yeast 7 g

Directions:
1. Mix the flour, yeast and salt in a large bowl.
2. Pour in 175 ml of hot water and oil.
3. Mix everything well. The dough should move away from the walls of the bowl.
4. Put the dough on the table, sprinkled with flour. Stir for 5 minutes.

5. Sprinkle cornmeal over the baking tray. Form a ball out of dough.
6. Put on a large baking sheet. Cover with a transparent pellicle and let stand for 15 minutes.
7. Roll out the dough. Lift the edges of the dough up, bend, to get a side.
8. Put the pizza base on the barbecue grill.
9. Fry over medium heat for 2-5 minutes until the bottom of the pizza is Golden.
10. Turn the base with tongs. Lightly brush with olive oil.
11. Sprinkle with mozzarella, then Basil and place the tomato slices on top.
12. Fry for another 3-5 minutes until the cheese starts to melt.
13. Sprinkle the remaining olive oil on the finished pizza. Sprinkle with salt and pepper.

Pizza With Onion And Asparagus

Ingredients:

- 85 gr. Fontana cheese, minced
- 1 tablespoon finely grated Pecorino cheese
- 1 tsp. leaf oregano, to break
- Salt and freshly ground pepper
- 6 pieces of thin asparagus
- 3 leeks
- 2 tsp olive oil
- 340 gr. pizza dough

Directions:

1. Light the grill. Mix asparagus and leek with 1 teaspoon of olive oil, season with salt and pepper.
2. Fry the vegetables on the grill over medium high heat, turning once, for about 2 minutes, until lightly charred. Shift the vegetables on

the Board and cut across into 2.5-centimeter pieces.

3. Form a pizza cake about 0.3 cm thick on a lightly floured work surface on a lightly floured work surface .
4. Grate the cake on both sides with the remaining olive oil.
5. Fry the cake on the grill over medium heat, turning once, until crispy and slightly charred edges, for 2 minutes on each side.
6. Place the cake on the work surface, put asparagus, leeks and sprinkle with Fontana and Pecorino cheese.
7. Return the pizza to the grill, cover it with a lid and cook for about a minute until the cheese melts. Before serving, sprinkle the pizza with oregano and season with pepper.

Crispy Crust Dough

Ingredients:

- 2 teaspoons salt
- 1 1/2 cups 110 degree water
- 2 1/2 tablespoons olive oil, divided
- 3 1/2 cups bread flour
- 1 teaspoon sugar
- 1 envelope dry yeast, instant variety

Directions:

1. In a mixing bowl, mix together the sugar, yeast, salt and bread flour.
2. With the mixer on, add the water and 2 tablespoons of the olive oil; beat until a dough ball is formed.
3. Add more flour by the tablespoon if the dough is sticky; add a little more water if it is too dry.

4. Form a ball out of the dough, put it on a floured surface and knead for about 3 minutes or until it is smooth and firm.
5. Use the remaining olive oil to grease the inside of another bowl; place the dough in it and turn to coat.
6. Let rise for 1 hour or until the dough doubles in size.
7. Turn the dough onto a floured surface and divide into 2 pieces to make 2 pizzas.
8. Cover with plastic wrap and let it rest for 10 minutes.

No-Rise Pizza Dough

Ingredients:

- 1 teaspoon salt
- 1 tablespoon sugar (white)
- 1 cup water at 110 degrees
- 3 cups all-purpose flour, not self-rising
- 1 package (1/4 ounce) dry yeast
- 2 tablespoons olive oil

Directions:

1. Combine all the dry Ingredients: in a bowl. Using your hands, mix in the oil and the water until a dough forms.
2. With floured hands, spread out the dough on a pizza or other pan.
3. Top as desired and bake at 375 for 20 minutes or until done.

Fast Pizza For Baking

Ingredients:

The dough for the base:

- 0.5 tsp baking powder
- 350 g of flour (2.5 cups)
- 0.5 tsp salt
- 250 g of thick cream
- 4 tbsp. milk
- 6 tbsp. vegetable oil

Filling:

- 3 not too sharp bitter pepper (optional)
- 15 button mushrooms, chopped
- Dried oregano (optional)
- Garlic salt (optional)
- 400 g grated cheese

- 0.5 cups of tomato sauce (or is diluted with water. Paste)
- 4 tomatoes, chopped
- a few slices of ham, sausage

Directions:
1. Mix all the Ingredients: for the dough. Baking lay baking paper.
2. Roll out the dough (fairly thin) and transfer to a baking sheet (it is convenient to the rolling pin).
3. Then you can distribute the dough a little more on the baking sheet with his hands. Prick with a fork in several places.
4. Heat oven to 200 C. The basis of grease tomato sauce, top with stuffing.
5. Season with oregano, garlic seasoning or any other seasoning to taste.
6. At the end sprinkle with grated cheese.
7. Bake in preheated oven for 25 minutes.

Quick Pizza Dough

Ingredients:

- 2.5 cups (350g) plain flour or bread
- 2 tbsp. vegetable oil
- 1 tsp salt
- 2 tsp (7 g), dry yeast
- 1 tsp Sahara
- 1 cup (250 ml), warm water (45 C)

Directions:

1. Preheat oven to 230 C. In a small bowl, dissolve yeast and sugar in warm (not hot!) Water.
2. Let stand 10 minutes to wake up the yeast and began to play.
3. Add flour, salt and oil and knead until you have a uniform dough. Give the dough for 5 minutes.

4. Baking tray or pizza stone to lightly greased and sprinkled with semolina or corn grits.
5. Put the dough on a floured table. Roll or shape hands flat cake.
6. Transfer the dough to a baking sheet.
7. Add the stuffing and bake in a well-heated oven (230 C) 15 20 minutes, or until lightly browned. Writing 5 minutes pizza cool before being cut.

Pizza Fruit Pizza

Ingredients:

For the Crust:

- 3/4 cup honey
- 1 teaspoon pure vanilla extract
- 1/2 teaspoon ground cinnamon
- 1/8 teaspoon salt
- 2 cups old fashioned oats
- ¾ cup oat flour I used Bob's Red Mill or you can make your own
- 3 tablespoons coconut oil room temperature (melted butter can be substituted)

For the Yogurt Filling:

- 1-2 tablespoons maple syrup or honey depending on your preference
- 1 teaspoon pure vanilla extract

- 1 1 1/3 cups plain Greek yogurt Thick, full-fat works best or use a non-dairy if needed(half yogurt and half softened cream cheese can also be substituted)

For the Fruit Topping:

- 1 medium kiwi sliced
- 2 large strawberries sliced
- 1/3 cup blueberries
- Plus any other fruits you like
- 1/2 cup blackberries
- 1/2 cup raspberries
- 1/3 cup mandarin oranges

Directions:
1. Preheat oven to 350 F.
2. Grease a 10-inch cake pan with baking spray or line with parchment paper and set aside.
3. In a large bowl, combine oats, oat flour, cinnamon, vanilla and salt together. Add the

honey and coconut oil and mix until dough is combined and sticks together. Use your hands or a fork as needed.
4. Spread the mixture into prepared pan and press down firmly with a spatula or the bottom of a glass cup.
5. Bake in preheated oven for 10 minutes. Remove from oven and allow to cool completely (place in the refrigerator or freezer to cool faster).
6. Meanwhile, in a medium mixing bowl, combine yogurt with honey and vanilla. Use an offset spatula to spread yogurt over cooled crust.
7. Decorate with your favorite combination of fruit. Enjoy immediately or place in the fridge to cool and set.

Pizza Stuff Crust Chipotle Chicken Pizza

Ingredients:

Pizza dough

- 1 tsp golden caster sugar
- 5.75 floz warm water
- 2 cups strong white bread flour
- 1 tsp salt
- 0.12 oz fast action yeast

Pizza sauce

- 14 oz tin Chopped Tomatoes
- 3 tbsp Tomato Puree
- 2 tbsp Chipotle Paste
- 3 tbsp Olive Oil
- 1 Onion chopped
- 3 Cloves Garlic crushed

For the Toppings

- 3.53 oz Cooked Chicken shredded
- 1 Yellow Pepper sliced
- 1 small Red Onion sliced
- 5.29 oz Mozzarella cut into strips (for stuffed crust)
- 3.53 oz Mozzarella sliced (for topping)

Directions:
1. Make the dough. Mix the flour, yeast and salt together in a large bowl.
2. Mix together the sugar and warm water then make a well in the centre of the dry Ingredients:.
3. Pour the sugar and water into the well.
4. Gradually mix the wet and dry Ingredients: together and then turn out onto a floured work surface. Knead for 10 minutes.
5. Flour the outside of the ball of dough then place in an oiled bowl.

6. At this stage you can either prove for about 15 minutes somewhere warm or put it into the fridge until you're ready to use.
7. Preheat the oven to 200° C. Make the sauce. Heat the olive oil over a medium heat.
8. Add the onion, garlic, plenty of salt and 40ml of water.
9. Once the water has evaporated pour in the tin of tomatoes and cook down until it's almost dry.
10. Mix in the tomato puree and chipotle paste and leave to cook a little more until it has a thick consistency.
11. Tip out onto a plate and allow to cool.
12. Split the dough in half and roll each ball of dough out into a circle.
13. Place on trays and spread the strips of mozzarella around the outer edge of the pizza making sure to leave a little gap at the edge.

14. Carefully fold the dough over the cheese and tuck in tightly pressing to seal. Repeat with the second pizza.
15. Spread the sauce around the middle of each pizza and split all the toppings between the two pizzas.
16. Bake for 15 minutes until all the cheese is melted.

Bacon Weave Pizza

Ingredients:

- 1 cup sliced green bell pepper
- 1/4 medium red onion , sliced
- 1/4 cup sliced black olives
- 1/4 cup grated parmesan
- 12 slices thick-cut bacon
- 1/2 cup pizza sauce
- 1 cup shredded mozzarella

Directions:

1. Preheat oven to 400°. Line a sizable baking sheet pan with parchment paper.
2. To create a bacon weave, line six bacon slices side-by-side on the baking sheet.
3. Lift up and fold back almost every other bacon slice, then lay a seventh slice at the top in the guts.

4. Lay folded-back slices along with seventh slice, then fold back the alternate slices.
5. Place eighth slice at the top, next to the seventh slice, weaving as if you did before.
6. Continue doing this process four more times to complete the weave.
7. Place an inverted, oven-proof cooling rack along with the bacon slices.
8. This can help them stay flat. Bake 23 to 25 minutes, or until bacon starts to crisp.
9. Remove baking sheet from oven and pour off as much fat since you can.
10. Carefully remove rack, then spread with pizza sauce leaving 1/2-inch roughly for crust.
11. Top with mozzarella, pepper, onions, olives, and Parmesan.
12. Return sheet to oven and continue baking until cheese is melty, another ten minutes.

Ban Mi Pizza

Ingredients:

- 1/2 fresh jalapeño, seeded and thinly sliced
- 12 ounces fresh deli whole-wheat pizza dough
- 1/2 teaspoon reduced-sodium soy sauce or tamari
- 1 1/2 tablespoons sesame oils, divided
- 5 ounces part-skim mozzarella cheese, shredded (about 1 1/4 cups)
- 1 1/2 tablespoons canola mayonnaise
- 1/2 teaspoon sriracha chili sauce
- 1/2 cup loosely packed fresh cilantro leaves
- 1 cup apple cider vinegar
- 1 cup water
- 1/2 cup granulated sugar
- 1/2 teaspoon kosher salt

- 1 cup matchstick-cut carrot
- 1/2 english cucumber, thinly sliced
- 1/3 cup thinly sliced radishes

Directions:
1. Place a pizza stone or baking sheet in oven.
2. Preheat oven to 500°F. (Usually do not remove pizza stone while oven preheats.)
3. Combine vinegar, 1 cup water, sugar, and salt in a saucepan. Bring to a simmer over medium-high; cook, stirring occasionally, until sugar and salt dissolve.
4. Stir in carrots, cucumber, radishes, and jalapeño. Remove from heat; let stand ten minutes. Drain and reserve.
5. Roll dough right into a 13-inch circle on a sizable little bit of parchment paper; pierce well with a fork. Brush soy sauce and 1 tablespoon sesame oil over dough.
6. Place dough (in some recoverable format) on preheated stone.

7. Bake at 500°F for 6 minutes.
8. Sprinkle mozzarella evenly over dough. Bake at 500°F for five minutes.
9. Combine mayonnaise, Sriracha, and remaining 1 1/2 teaspoons sesame oil.
10. Spread pickled vegetables evenly over pizza. Drizzle mayonnaise mixture over top. Sprinkle with cilantro. Cut into 8 slices.

Vegetarian Minestrone Soup

Ingredients:

- ¼ cup celery
- 2 tablespoons basil
- 1/3 tsp oregano
- ¼ tsp black pepper
- 1 can plum tomatoes
- 2 cloves garlic
- ½ cup uncooked pasta
- 1 tablespoon olive oil
- ¾ cup onion
- 2 ½ cups water
- 2 cups zucchini
- 1 cup sliced carrots
- 1 cup beans

Directions:

1. In a saucepan add oil, onion and sauté for 4-5 minutes
2. Add remaining Ingredients: and bring to a boil
3. Reduce heat and simmer on low heat for 20-25 minutes
4. Add pasta and cook until pasta is al dente for 10-12 minutes
5. When ready, remove from heat and serve

Cabbage Stew

Ingredients:

- 1 onion
- 2 cloves garlic
- 2 tablespoons aminos
- 4 cups chicken stock
- 1 lb. bison
- 1 tablespoon olive oil
- ¼ cabbage
- 2 carrots

Directions:

1. In a pot sauté the carrot, onion and cabbage for 2-3 minutes
2. Add bison and cook for 4-5 minutes
3. Add chicken stock, garlic, ginger and coconut aminos
4. Cook for 25-30 minutes

5. When ready from heat garnish with pepper and serve

Pizza With Prosciutto And Tomatoes

Ingredients:

Pizza dough

- 2 tsp chopped garlic
- Two 400-gram jars of chopped tomatoes, dry
- 1/2 Cup Basil leaves, tear into small pieces
- 12 slices of prosciutto, torn into large pieces
- 230 gr. Fontana cheese, minced
- 1/2 Cup grated Pecorino Romano cheese
- Olive oil

Directions:

1. Light the grill. Place the grid in 7.5-10 cm from the coals. mix Fontana cheese and Romano Pecorino in a medium bowl.
2. Roll out a thin pellet with a thickness of about 0.2 cm Greased with olive oil and lay out on the net.

3. Cook for a minute until bubbles and grill marks begin to appear.
4. Turn the cake over and cook for another 30-40 seconds. Grease the top side of the cake with olive oil and turn over.
5. Sprinkle the cake with garlic, cheese, sliced tomatoes.
6. Sprinkle 1/2 tablespoon of olive oil. Place the pizza on the grill in the indirect heating zone.
7. Periodically, use the tongs to rotate the pizza and make sure that it is not burnt from the bottom.
8. Cook for about 3-4 minutes.
9. Sprinkle the pizza with Basil leaves and place the prosciutto, About a minute before the end of cooking.
10. When the cheese melts, and the tomatoes warm up and become soft enough — the pizza is ready.

Pizza With Cheese And Pesto

Ingredients:

- 1/2 Cup olive oil
- 1/2 Cup grated Parmigianino cheese
- 1 Cup of mozzarella, divided into small pieces
- 1/2 Cup Fontana cheese
- 1/2 Cup Provolone cheese
- 450 gr. pizza dough
- 1/2 Cup unsalted roasted pistachios
- 2 small garlic cloves
- 2 cups baby arugula
- 1 Cup Basil leaves
- 1/2 teaspoon chopped red pepper
- Salt and freshly ground black pepper

Directions:

1. For the pesto: grind the pistachios and garlic in a food processor. Then add arugula, Basil, red pepper and grind again. Pour 1/2 Cup olive oil slowly without turning off the combine. Add Parmigianino and mix it all together again. Salt and pepper.
2. Light the grill, put the mozzarella, Fontana and Provolone cheese in a bowl. The dough is divided into 4 parts. Form a dough 25-centimeter cake 0.3 cm thick on a lightly floured work surface. Oil it.
3. Fry the tortilla on the grill over medium high heat, turning once until it is slightly charred, about 4 minutes.
4. Put the cake to the work surface. Grease pesto, sprinkle with cheese, salt and pepper.
5. Again put on the grill and cook for about 4 minutes on a moderately low heat under the lid until the cheese melts.

Spicy Pizza With Sausages

Ingredients:

- Pinch of sugar
- 230 gr. mozzarella, finely chopped
- 2 sausages
- 4 pepper oscine red pepper, remove seeds and thinly slice
- Basil leaves for decoration
- 450 gr. for pizza dough
- 450 gr. squash pumpkin, grate on a grater with large holes
- 1/2 tsp salt + for seasoning
- 2 tbsp of olive oil
- One 400-gram jar of chopped tomatoes, dry

Directions:

1. Light the grill. put the squash in a colander, set over a medium bowl, season 1/2 teaspoon of salt, let stand for 15 minutes, then squeeze out excess water.
2. Heat 2 tablespoons of olive oil in a large frying pan, add the courgettes and cook until Golden brown for about 3 minutes.
3. Fry the sausages on the grill, allow to cool slightly, then thinly cut into slices.
4. Turn the tomatoes in a blender, season with salt and pepper sauce. Form a 0.6 cm thick pizza pie on a lightly floured work surface.
5. Grease with olive oil, put on a greased grill. Simmer until the dough is left on the grill for about 3 minutes. Put the cake on a baking sheet, grease with olive oil.
6. Grease the cake with cooked tomato sauce, retreating 2 cm from the edge. Spread on a tortilla zucchini, mozzarella cheese and sauce on top.

7. Put the pizza on the grill, close and cook for 4-5 minutes until the cheese melts.
8. Put the pizza on a plate, sprinkle with pepper online and Basil leaves and serve immediately.

Mama's Best Crust

Ingredients:

- 2 cups bread flour
- 2 tablespoons olive oil
- 1 teaspoon kosher salt
- 2 teaspoons sugar
- 1 cup warm water, 110 degrees
- 1 package (1/4 ounce) active dry yeast

Directions:

1. Dissolve the yeast in the water and let stand for 10 minutes or until creamy.
2. Combine the flour, olive oil, sugar, salt and yeast mixture in a large bowl; beat until a stiff dough results.
3. Cover with a damp cloth or plastic wrap and let rise for 30 minutes or until double in size.

4. Put the dough on a floured surface and roll or push into a pizza shape that fits the pan being used.
5. Top with desired toppings; bake at 350 for about 20 minutes.

Honey And Whole Wheat Dough

Ingredients:

- 1/4 cup wheat germ, dry
- 1 teaspoon salt
- 1 tablespoon natural honey
- 1 package (.25 ounce) dry yeast, active
- 1 cup 110 degree water
- 2 cups flour, whole wheat variety (bread flour is best)

Directions:
1. Preheat the oven to 350 degrees.
2. Sprinkle 1 teaspoon dry cornmeal over a pizza pan surface to prevent the crust from sticking to it.
3. Dissolve the yeast in the water until foamy/creamy, about 10 minutes.

4. Combine the dry Ingredients: in a bowl; make a hole in the middle and add the honey and the yeast mixture.
5. Stir well with a fork until completely combined.
6. Cover and let rise for no more than 30 minutes.
7. Push the dough out to the shape of the pizza pan and use a fork to poke a few holes in it – this will prevent an uneven crust.
8. Bake for 7 minutes in the oven or 10 minutes if a more crispy crust is preferred.

Pizza Dough In The Bread Maker

Ingredients:

- 300 g of flour (2 1/2 cups)
- 2 tsp Sahara
- 2 tsp dry yeast
- 200 ml of warm water
- 3/4 tsp salt
- 2 tbsp. olive oil

Directions:
1. Add the Ingredients: in the order specified by the manufacturer.
2. Turn the dough mode and start the cycle.
3. When the time has elapsed, remove the dough.
4. Put the dough in a greased form and spread on the bottom.

5. Let stand for 10 minutes. Preheat oven to 200 C.
6. Put the dough on top of the pizza sauce and toppings. Top -The raw material.
7. Bake 15 20 minutes, or until lightly browned basis.

Pizza Minute

Ingredients:

Pizza dough:

- 4 tbsp. mayonnaise
- 2/3 cups flour (8-10 tbsp. without slides)
- a pinch of salt
- 2 eggs
- 4 tbsp. sour cream

Pizza toppings:

- 100 g of sausage or ham
- 100 g of cheese
- Ketchup, mayonnaise
- 1 tomato

Directions:

1. Prepare the batter: Beat eggs slightly, add the sour cream and mayonnaise, mix well.

2. Gradually add the flour; the dough should get watery, like thick cream.
3. The dough can be added a pinch of salt and sugar.
4. For the filling just cut tomato slices, ham or sausage subtly. You can take the fresh herbs and olives.
5. The pan well warm assurances fire oiled.
6. Pour a thin layer of dough and immediately reduce the heat to a small.
7. If you have a small frying pan, it is best to divide the dough into 2 parts.
8. Coat the dough on top of ketchup and mayonnaise, put slices of tomato, then a ham or sausage.
9. Sprinkle with cheese.
10. The pan cover and cook a few minutes until the cheese melts.
11. If you are not well melted cheese, then check out the cake when it is ready, increase the

heat to high for a couple of seconds, then immediately turn off the heat and leave the pizza for a few minutes under the lid.

Home Fast Pizza

Ingredients:

Pizza dough:

- 2 eggs
- 4 tbsp. sour cream
- 5 tbsp. mayonnaise
- 10 tbsp. flour without slides
- a pinch of salt

Pizza toppings:

- Salami or sausage
- 100 g of cheese
- Ketchup, mayonnaise
- 1 tomato

Directions:

1. Prepare the batter: Beat eggs slightly, add the sour cream and mayonnaise, mix well.

2. According spoon add the flour.
3. Depending on how thick cream and mayonnaise, flour may be less or more.
4. I used a very thick mayonnaise and sour cream.
5. Is mixed into the flour gradually need to make the dough has turned watery (like on pancakes) with no lumps.
6. Baking pan greased with oil well, pour a thin layer of batter. I usually divide the dough into 2 pizza, because the form is not large.
7. Coat the dough on top of ketchup, if you want you can even lubricate and mayonnaise.
8. Top with tomato slices and salami.
9. Sprinkle with grated cheese. I just planed cheese knife.
10. Put the pizza in the oven. Bake at 220 C for about 10 minutes until the pizza is golden brown.

Pizza Roasted Garlic And Mushroom Pizza

Ingredients:

- ¼ tsp each: salt, pepper, dried basil, onion powder
- 3 TBS Parmesan
- 1 whole wheat pizza dough
- 1 cup mozzarella cheese, shredded
- ½ cup Parmigiano-Reggiano, grated
- 2 TBS minced fresh herbs such as parsley
- 6 garlic cloves (unpeeled!)
- splash olive oil
- 8 oz mushrooms, sliced
- 1 tsp white wine vinegar
- 1 TBS each: butter and all purpose flour
- ½ cup milk of choice

Directions:

1. Preheat oven to 400 F.
2. Toss unpeeled garlic with a splash of olive oil. Wrap in a piece of foil. Roast garlic in the preheated oven for 40 minutes.
3. Meanwhile, prep your pizza dough.
4. Add mushrooms to a large skillet and cook over medium heat until the liquid is released and evaporated. Stir in white wine vinegar and set aside.
5. In another small skillet, whisk together butter and flour over medium heat. Let this mixture bubble for 1 minutes, stirring constantly. Whisk in milk, and stir until thickened.
6. Mix salt, pepper, basil, onion powder, and Parmesan.
7. Peel roasted garlic and add to the sauce. Transfer to a mini food processor or use a hand blender to blend the garlic cloves into the sauce. Set white sauce aside.

8. Increase oven temperature to 425 F.
9. Press dough out into a 12 inch circle. Spread white sauce evenly over dough. Top with mozzarella, parmigiano-reggiano, and sautéed mushrooms.
10. Bake in the preheated oven (preferably on a pizza stone) for 12 minutes, or until the cheese is starting to turn golden brown.
11. Top with herbs, and cut into 6 slices.

Pizza Grilled Prosciutto, Spinach, And Burrito Pizza

Ingredients:

Pizza dough

- Spinach
- Mozzarella, shredded
- Burrata (an italian milk cheese)
- Cornmeal
- Tomato sauce (see recipe below)
- Prosciutto

For the Tomato Sauce

- 1 28 ounce can crushed tomatoes
- ½ onion
- 1 teaspoon kosher salt
- 4 tablespoons unsalted butter

Directions:

For tomato sauce

1. Place all Ingredients: into a small sauce pan. Bring to a simmer and cook, uncovered, for 40 minutes.
2. Stir occasionally to prevent burning. Use immediately or store in an airtight container in the fridge for 1 week or the freezer for 3 months.

For pizza

1. Roll out the dough on a lightly floured surface according to the Directions:. Place a thin layer of tomato sauce and mozzarella onto the top of the pizza.
2. Place the pizza stones onto the grill (or oven). Heat the grill (or oven) to 500 degrees. Place the pizza onto the stones and close the lid. Grill for about 4 minutes, or until the crust begins to brown (be sure to monitor the bottom of the pizza, it can burn quickly).

3. Top the pizza with small bite-sized portions of prosciutto. Return the pizza to the grill and cook for 30 seconds. Remove from the heat once again and add a handful of spinach. Place back onto the grill and let cook for 30 seconds.
4. Remove the pizza from the grill and add the burrata onto the pizza. Serve immediately.

Pizza Grilled Strawberry Balsamic Herb Pizza

Ingredients:

- 1/2 cup fresh watercress, divided
- 4 ounces fresh, crumbled goat cheese
- 1/2 cup balsamic vinegar glaze
- 3 Tablespoons fresh basil leaves, roughly torn
- 1 Tablespoon fresh mint leaves, roughly torn
- Kosher salt to taste
- 1 ball of pizza dough, rolled thin
- 1/4 cup cornmeal for dusting
- 1 Tablespoon extra virgin olive oil
- 1 pint fresh strawberries, hulled and thinly sliced

Directions:

1. Add Kettle Pizza insert to grill according to manufacturer Directions:. Arrange charcoal in

kettle grill according to Directions: and allow charcoal to come up to temperature.
2. Place a large sheet of parchment paper on a pizza peel and dust generously with cornmeal.
3. Roll pizza dough to 1/8" thickness on a lightly floured surface and transferred to cornmeal dusted parchment.
4. Brush olive oil in an even layer over the surface of the dough.
5. Spread strawberry slices in an even layer over pizza.
6. Add an even layer of watercress and goat cheese over pizza.
7. When grill is ready, slide pizza, with parchment paper onto pizza stone on grill.
8. Bake for one minute before carefully removing parchment (transferring with parchment is easier than moving raw dough alone).

9. Bake pizza for 3 to 5 minutes, according to Kettle Pizza Directions:, until crust is crisp and toppings are golden. If needed, use pizza peel to lift pizza into upper dome of grill for one minute to cook toppings evenly.
10. Remove pizza from oven and garnish generously with balsamic glaze, fresh mint and basil and Kosher salt before serving.

Bbq Chicken Crust Pizza

Ingredients:

- 1/4 cup barbecue sauce
- 1 cup shredded gouda
- 1/3 cup sliced red onion
- 2 tablespoons sliced green onions
- Ranch dressing, for drizzling
- 1 pound. Ground chicken
- 1 1/2 cups. Shredded mozzarella
- 1 teaspoon garlic powder
- Kosher salt
- Freshly ground black pepper

Directions:

1. Preheat oven to 400º and line a baking sheet with parchment paper. In a huge bowl, stir together ground chicken, 1/2 cup mozzarella,

and garlic powder and season with salt and pepper.
2. Spray the prepared baking sheet as well as your hands with cooking spray.
3. Form chicken mixture into pizza "crusts." Bake until chicken is cooked through and golden, 20 to 22 minutes.
4. Remove from oven and heat broiler.
5. Spread a thin layer of barbecue sauce on pizza crusts and top with remaining 1 cup mozzarella and Gouda.
6. Top with red and green onions and drizzle with an increase of barbecue sauce.
7. Broil until cheese is melty, three minutes. Drizzle with ranch dressing and serve.

Bbq Chicken Pizza

Ingredients:

- 1/4 medium red onion , thinly sliced
- 1/3 cup shredded gouda
- Pinch crushed red pepper flakes (optional)
- 2 tablespoons freshly chopped cilantro
- 1 pound . Refrigerated pizza dough, divided into 2 pieces
- 2 cups cooked shredded chicken
- 3/4 cup barbecue sauce , divided
- 1 cup shredded mozzarella

Directions:

1. Preheat oven to 500°.
2. Line two large baking sheets with parchment paper and grease with cooking spray.
3. In a medium bowl, stir together chicken and 1/4 cup barbecue sauce.

4. On a lightly floured surface, roll out pizza dough into a sizable circle, then slide onto prepared baking sheet.
5. Top each pizza with 1/4 cup barbecue sauce, then half the chicken mixture, spreading within an even layer and leaving 1" around the edge bare.
6. Next add a straight layer of mozzarella and red onion, then top with gouda.
7. Sprinkle with crushed red pepper flakes if using. Bake until cheese is melty and dough is cooked through, 20 to 25 minutes.
8. Garnish with cilantro before serving.

Bbq Chicken Pizza Sliders

Ingredients:

- 1/4 cup freshly chopped cilantro
- 3 slices cheddar
- 1/4 cup butter
- 1 clove garlic , minced
- 1 teaspoon onion powder
- 12 Hawaiian rolls
- 3 cups shredded rotisserie chicken
- 1/2 cup barbecue sauce
- 1/4 cup diced red onion

Directions:

1. Preheat oven to 350º. Slice slider rolls in two and place underneath halves in a 9"-x-13" baking dish.

2. In a big bowl, add shredded chicken and barbecue sauce and stir to coat.
3. Spoon chicken over the slider rolls and sprinkle with red onion and cilantro.
4. Cut each slice of cheese into 4 pieces and top each slider with cheese.
5. Place top of slider rolls over the sandwiches.
6. Place butter in a microwave-safe bowl and heat on low until melted, 30 seconds.
7. Add garlic and onion powder and stir.
8. Brush the tops of the sliders with garlic butter, then cover the dish tightly with foil and bake, 15 minutes.

Chicken Rice Soup

Ingredients:

- 2 cloves garlic
- 6 cups chicken broth
- ½ cup brown rice
- ¼ cup lemon juice
- 1 tsp black pepper
- ¼ cup parsley
- 1 tablespoon olive oil
- 1 cup carrot
- 1 cup onion
- 1 cup celery
- 1 chicken breast

Directions:

1. In a pot sauté the carrot, onion and celery for 2-3 minutes

2. Add chicken breast and cook for another 4-5 minutes
3. Add rice, lemon juice, pepper and chicken broth
4. Cook for 30-40 minutes on high heat
5. When soup is cooked remove from heat
6. Garnish with parsley and serve

Miso Soup

Ingredients:

- 2 tablespoons miso paste
- 10 oz. codfish fillet
- 2 cups vegetables
- ¼ cup broccoli sprouts
- 1 tablespoon scallion
- 1 tablespoon olive oil
- 2 tablespoons arame
- 1 cup water
- 2 cups chicken broth
- 1 cup mushrooms

Directions:
1. In a bowl soak arame and set aside
2. In a saucepan add broth and bring to a boil
3. Add the cod to the saucepan, vegetables. cover and cook for 5-6 minutes

4. Stir in the miso paste and cook until soup is ready
5. Ladle into bowls top with scallions and serve

Grilled Pizza From Mario Batali

Ingredients:

- 1/2 cup black pitted black olives, chopped
- 2 cups of tomato sauce
- 230 gr. mozzarella, coarsely chopped
- 1/2 cup basil leaves
- 1/2 cup pine nuts
- 230 gr. Fontana cheese, coarsely chopped
- Salt Malden.

Directions:

1. Light the grill. When the coals are ready, move 2/3 to one side and leave the rest to the other, thus creating two heating zones.
2. Fry pine nuts until Golden brown for about 1 minute in a small iron pan.
3. Form a 25-centimeter flat cake on a lightly oiled baking sheet.

4. Place the tortilla on the grill in a hotter place.
5. Cook for about 1 minute until there are marks on the grill.
6. Use the tongs to move the cake to another heating zone and continue cooking for about 2 minutes until the cake is Golden brown and covered with bubbles.
7. Turn the cake over and return to a hotter place.
8. Cook for a minute, then move to another area.
9. Lubricate the cake with tomato sauce, sprinkle mozzarella.
10. Close the grill and cook for about 2 minutes until it melts.
11. Put the pizza on a cutting Board, decorate with Basil leaves and sprinkle with Malden salt.

12. Cook the cake in the same way, sprinkle cheese Fontana olives and pine nuts at the end.
13. Cook under a closed lid for about 2 minutes until the cheese melts.
14. Cut into pieces and serve immediately. Repeat with the rest of the other pellet

Pizza Bbq Chicken

Ingredients:

- 2/3 tbsp. (90 gr.) grated smoked Gouda cheese
- 2/3 tbsp. (90 gr.) grated mozzarella cheese
- 1/2 small head of red onion, cut into thin rings
- Fresh coriander leaves
- 1 tbsp olive oil, plus more for greasing
- 250 grams. finished pizza dough, room temperature
- 1/3 tbsp. and 2 tbsp. dark barbecue sauce
- 250 gr. chicken breast fillet without skin
- Salt and freshly ground pepper

Directions:
1. Place the baking sheet in the upper part of the oven and heat at 220°C. for 30 Minutes.

2. Grease the parchment paper with olive oil.
3. Put the dough on parchment paper and form hands in a round layer with a diameter of 25 cm.
4. Spread the dough with olive oil, cover with another sheet of parchment paper.
5. Leave the dough to rise, for 30 minutes.
6. Mix in a small bowl 2 tbsp barbecue sauce and 1 tsp olive oil.
7. Place the chicken breast in a baking dish, salt, pepper and grate with a mixture of barbecue sauce.
8. Bake the chicken breast in the middle of the oven for 20 minutes. Cool, then cut the meat into cubes.
9. Uncover the dough and spread 1/3 Cup barbecue sauce, leaving 2 cm on each side.
10. Lay on top layers of chicken, Gouda, mozzarella and red onion.

11. Put the pizza with parchment paper onto the hot baking tray and bake until the cheese has melted and the cake will not become Golden brown, 20 to 25 minutes.

12. Sprinkle the pizza with the cilantro leaves.

Pizza With Grilled Vegetables

Ingredients:

- Warm water 225 ml
- Olive oil 2 tbsp
- Flour 300 g
- Salt pinch
- Dry yeast 6 g

For filling:

- Mozzarella 1 pc
- Tomato sauce 2-3 tbsp
- Zucchini 1/2 pc

Directions:

1. Mix flour, salt and yeast. Connect oil and water in a separate container . Pour the liquid into the flour mixture and knead the dough.

Put to the table, sprinkled with flour and knead the dough for 2-3 minutes.
2. Put the dough in a bowl and grease with olive oil. Cover the bowl with cling pellicle and put in a warm place for 30-40 minutes, or until the dough has increased in volume 2 times.
3. Then again, you need to knead in for 1-2 minutes. Roll out the dough in a circle on a floured surface and put on a greased baking sheet. Make a small dough and fill with filling.
4. Prepare the filling. Cut the vegetables into slices. Break the slices of Mozzarella.
5. Fold all the vegetables in a form, sprinkle with olive oil and season to taste. Bake in the grill at a temperature of 200 C 25-30 minutes.
6. Lubricate the basis of the tomato sauce, arrange slices of vegetables and mozzarella on top . Send in a preheated 200 C oven for 15-20 minutes. Decorate the finished pizza with a sprig of rosemary and serve.

Master Pizza Dough

Ingredients:

- 1 cup 120 degree water
- 2 tablespoons olive oil
- 1 teaspoon cornmeal to sprinkle on pizza pan
- 2 1/2 cups all-purpose flour, maybe a little more, if needed
- 1 packet rapid rise yeast (1/4 ounce size)
- 3/4 teaspoon salt

Directions:
1. Combine the flour, dry yeast and salt in a large bowl; stir in the water and olive oil, adding additional flour if needed to form a soft dough.
2. Turn the dough onto a floured surface and knead for 6 minutes or until smooth.

3. Cover and let the dough rest for 10 minutes to rise slightly.
4. Spray oil onto the size pizza pans being used and sprinkle the cornmeal over the pan surface. Shape the dough onto the pan(s) and top as desired.
5. Preheat the oven to 400 degrees and bake the pizza(s) for 20 – 30 minutes depending on whether you are cooking 1 thick or 2 thin pizzas.

Rye Dough

Ingredients:

- 1 1/2 cups room temperature water, divided
- 1 teaspoon dark brown sugar
- 1 package dry yeast, active (1/4 ounce)
- 2 tablespoons olive oil
- 2 1/2 cups all-purpose flour, unbleached
- 1 cup rye flour, lightly sifted
- 1 teaspoon kosher salt

Directions:

1. Mix together the all-purpose and rye flours with the salt in a mixing bowl.
2. Heat 1/2 cup of water in the microwave for 30 seconds; stir the brown sugar and yeast into the water and stir until dissolved. Let the mixture stand for 10 minutes; pour into the mixed flour.

3. Heat the remaining 1 cup of water for 30 seconds; add the olive oil to the water and stir. Add to the flour mixture and stir to form a dough. If needed add either more flour or water to the mixture to form a firm dough.
4. Knead the dough in the bowl for 3 minutes; cover and let rise for 1 hour or until doubled in size, covered with a damp towel or plastic wrap.
5. Roll the dough out on a floured surface to fit the size pan being used.

Pizza With Sausage

Ingredients:

Pizza dough:

- 4-5 cups flour
- 1.5 tsp salt
- 2 tbsp. vegetable oil
- 1.5 cups of warm water
- 10 g of dry active yeast (3 tsp)

Pizza toppings:

- Cheese taste
- a bit of tomato sauce
- 300 g of sausages

Directions:
1. Dissolve yeast in water.
2. In a deep bowl, mix flour and salt. Add the yeast and knead the dough.

3. If the dough is too stiff, add a little water. Or conversely, if it is too liquid add the flour.
4. Turn dough out onto floured board and knead until it will gather into a ball, and is smooth and elastic.
5. Lubricate the plastic bowl with vegetable oil, put it in the dough and cover with cling film or a damp towel or.
6. Put the dough in a warm place hours 2. It must be doubled.
7. Now you can make a pizza. I love cake pizza average thickness.
8. From proportions, which I quoted above, it is possible to make three pizzas.
9. Roll out a third test. Put it on a greased round baking.
10. Grease a cake tomato sauce can be spread with mayonnaise.
11. Lay thin slices of sausage. Sprinkle with grated cheese.

12. Place the pizza in a preheated 200° C oven for about 15-20 minutes, until lightly browned edge.

The Dough For Pizza Without Yeast

Ingredients:

- 2/3 cup milk
- 2 tsp baking powder
- 2 cups of flour
- 1/3 cup vegetable oil
- a pinch of salt, basil, pepper

Directions:

1. The Ingredients: are mixed in a bowl manually until smooth. (The dough should have elastic and a little tight).
2. Roll out the dough (who he loves thick or thin), prick in several places with a fork.
3. Choose toppings to your taste. Oven for about 30 minutes at a temperature of 180° C.

Pizza Low Carb Crust Less Pizza

Ingredients:

- 2 Cups Cheese, shredded
- Pepperoni, sliced
- Seasonings, (optional) Oregano, garlic powder and dried basil
- Low Carb Pizza Sauce, (optional)

Directions:

1. In a nonstick skillet, add a thin and even layer of shredded cheese.
2. Top with whatever toppings you'd like.
3. Cover with a glass lid and cook until the cheese melts and the bottom and edges become golden.
4. Remove from heat and allow the cheese to cool before taking out of pan.
5. Cut into pizza slices and serve with your favorite dipping sauce!

Pizza Grilled Home Style Pizza With Honey Sriracha Glaze

Ingredients:

- ½ cup sliced mushrooms
- Fresh thyme leaves
- Salt and pepper
- Red chili flakes
- Greens
- Flour & Cornmeal
- 1 batch of store bought or homemade pizza dough
- ½ cup pizza sauce
- ½ cup cheese, grated
- ¼ cup pepperoni
- ¼ of a purple onion, thinly sliced

For the Sauce:

- ½-1 teaspoon Sriracha sauce
- 1 teaspoon honey

Directions:

1. Preheat grill and pizza stone.
2. Once grill is preheated (and not before!) dust dough and cutting board thoroughly with flour.
3. Press or roll dough to desired thickness turning frequently to be sure bottom is not sticking.
4. Sprinkle pizza peel heavily with cornmeal and transfer dough to peel.
5. Quickly add toppings and transfer to grill.
6. If you wait too long the dough will start to rise and will stick to peel and you will end up with a mess.
7. Cook to desired level of doneness (between 7-20 minutes depending on how hot you are able to get your grill).

8. The last 2 minutes of cooking brush on the sriracha honey glaze on crust if desired.
9. Top pizza with greens, red chili flakes and honey if desired.

Bbq Chicken Skillet Pizza

Ingredients:

- 2 tablespoons barbecue sauce , plus more for drizzling
- 1/2 cup shredded cheddar
- 1/2 cup shredded fontina
- 1/4 small red onion , thinly sliced
- ranch dressing, for drizzling
- freshly chopped chives , for garnish
- 1 tablespoon extra-virgin olive oil , plus more for brushing
- 1/2 pound . boneless skinless chicken breasts , cut into 1" pieces
- kosher salt
- freshly ground black pepper
- all-purpose flour , for dough

- 1 pound . pizza dough, at room temperature

Directions:
1. Preheat oven to 500°. In a huge skillet over medium-high heat, heat oil.
2. Add chicken and cook until golden no longer pink, 6 minutes per side.
3. Season generously with salt and pepper.
4. Meanwhile, brush an ovenproof skillet with oil.
5. On a floured work surface, roll out dough until circumference matches your skillet.
6. Transfer to skillet. Leaving a 1/2" border for the crust, spread barbecue sauce onto dough.
7. Top with cheddar, fontina, chicken, and red onion. Brush crust with essential olive oil and sprinkle with salt.
8. Bake until crust is crispy and cheese is melty, 23 to 25 minutes.
9. Drizzle with barbecue sauce and ranch and garnish with chives.

Bbq Pizza With Slaw Recipe

Ingredients:

- 3 ounces reduced-fat sharp cheddar cheese, grated (about 3/4 cup)
- 2 teaspoons cider vinegar
- 2 teaspoons extra-virgin olive oil
- dash of sugar
- 1/4 cup thinly sliced green cabbage
- 1/4 cup thinly sliced red onion
- 3 tablespoons grated carrots
- 2 tablespoons chopped fresh flat-leaf parsley
- 1/2 teaspoon crushed red pepper
- 12 ounces refrigerated fresh pizza dough
- 1/3 cup unsalted ketchup
- 1/4 cup lower-sodium marinara sauce
- 3 tablespoons water

- 1 tablespoon honey mustard
- 1 teaspoon ground ancho chile pepper
- 1 teaspoon lower-sodium worcestershire sauce
- 3/4 teaspoon smoked paprika
- 3/4 teaspoon garlic powder
- 1/2 teaspoon onion powder
- 3 ounces shredded skinless, boneless rotisserie chicken breast
- 2 teaspoons cornmeal

Directions:
1. Remove dough coming from the refrigerator. Let endure at room temp, covered, for half an hour.
2. Place a new pizza stone or perhaps heavy baking linen in oven.

3. Preset the oven to 500° (keep pizza natural stone or baking linen in the oven considering that it preheats).
4. Combine ketchup and after that 8 Ingredients: (through onion powder) within a tiny saucepan; provide a simmer.
5. Lessen heat; cook 6th minutes.
6. Combine a couple of tablespoons ketchup blend and chicken within a tiny bowl; throw out to coat.
7. Roll dough in a 14-inch circle over a lightly floured surface; pierce liberally with a fork.
8. Carefully remove pizza stone from oven. Sprinkle cornmeal over stone; place dough on stone.
9. Spread remaining sauce over crust, leaving a 1/2-inch border.
10. Arrange chicken mixture over dough. Sprinkle with cheese.

11. Bake at 500° for 9 minutes or until crust and cheese are browned.
12. Combine vinegar, oil, and sugar in a medium bowl, stirring with a whisk.
13. Stir in cabbage, onion, and carrot; toss to coat.
14. Top pizza with cabbage mixture, parsley, and red pepper. Cut into 8 wedges.

Grilled Pizza

Ingredients:

- White vinegar-1 teaspoon
- Extra virgin olive oil-2 tablespoons
- Garlic-3 cloves (finely chopped)
- Canned tomatoes-2 cups (finely chopped)
- Oregano-1 ½ teaspoons
- Dried Basil ¾ teaspoons
- Dried rosemary ¼ teaspoon
- Cumin ¼ teaspoon
- Dry yeast 2 ¼ teaspoons
- Sugar 2 teaspoons
- Warm water 1 ½ Cup
- Extra virgin olive oil-3 tablespoons + some more for lubrication
- Salt 1 ½ teaspoons

- Flour-3 ¾ 4 ¼ cups
- Salt and pepper – to taste

Directions:

1. Take ½ Cup water, add 2 teaspoons sugar and yeast and mix thoroughly to dissolve the yeast. Leave on for 5 minutes.
2. Pour the remaining glass of warm water, olive oil and vinegar, add salt.
3. Stirring with a mixer, pour half the flour slowly.
4. Stir until smooth and cover the remaining flour. Knead the dough: it should be elastic and not stick to the hands. Wrap the dough container in plastic wrap and leave in a warm place for 1.5-2 hours until it doubles in size.
5. Heat olive oil in a saucepan over medium-high heat for sauce . Add garlic to hot oil. Add all other Ingredients: and mix thoroughly. When the surface will appear to bubble reduce heat

to low. Cook the sauce for about 20 minutes, stirring occasionally.

6. Preheat the grill rack. Divide the dough into 6 equal parts. Roll out onto floured surface. Grease the grill rack and your pizzas with olive oil. Put the dough on the grates (oiled side down).

7. Hold on the grill for 2-3 minutes, oil the top part, turn over. Apply the sauce and put the filling. Keep on the grill for a few more minutes

Pizza Margarita With Two Grilled Cheeses

Ingredients:

- 6 tablespoons chopped tomatoes, canned in a thick puree
- 1/4 tablespoon olive oil
- 1/2 tsp crushed fresh garlic
- 8 Basil leaves
- 170 gr. pizza dough
- 1/2 tablespoon grated Fontina cheese (loosely compacted)
- 2 tablespoons grated Pecorino Romano cheese

Directions:

1. Prepare the charcoal grill by installing the grill at a distance of 8-10 cm above the coal.
2. Put the dough on a large, oiled inverted baking sheet and, stretching, form a circle of

his hands with a diameter of 25-30 cm and a thickness of 0.3 cm Do not make the bumpers.
3. You can also form a rectangle from the test, rather than a circle.
4. Form is not important, as long as the base has a uniform thickness.
5. When the grill warms up.
6. Pick up the loose end and stretch the remaining batter on the grate over the fire.
7. The dough will swell slightly in a minute, the sole will harden, and there will be characteristic strips from the grill.
8. Tongs immediately turn the base and shift to the coldest part of the grill.
9. Quickly lubricate the baked surface with olive oil. Sprinkle the base with garlic and cheese, put some tomatoes on the cheese.
10. Do not cover the entire surface of the pizza with tomatoes. Finally, pour 1-2 tablespoons of olive oil over the pizza.

11. Slide the pizza back into the hot part, but not directly over the coal.
12. Tongs often turn the pizza to different parts of it fell into a zone of extreme heat.
13. Often check the bottom of the pizza, so it is not burnt.
14. The pizza will be ready when the cheese melts on top and starts to bubble, after about 6-8 minutes.
15. Serve immediately, sprinkle with Basil leaves and sprinkle with olive oil again.

Grilled Avocado With Tomato Salsa

Ingredients:

- Oil (olive) 1 tablespoon
- Pepper (dried chili) ¼ tsp
- Lime (juice) to taste
- Pepper (black ground) to taste
- Salt to taste
- Avocado 2 PCs.
- Tomatoes 1 PCs.
- Bow (green) 1 quill
- Kinza 2 twigs

Directions:
1. Preheat the grill or prepare the coals.
2. Cut the tomatoes into cubes. Chop the greens.

3. Mix tomatoes and herbs, add chili, half a tablespoon of olive oil, lime juice and a little salt to taste.
4. Cut the avocado in half and remove the bone.
5. Lubricate each half of the avocado with olive oil and put on the grid. Cook for a few minutes.
6. Fill the avocado halves with tomato salsa and serve

Deep Dish Pizza Dough

Ingredients:

- 1/4 cup corn oil
- 2 teaspoons kosher salt
- 6 tablespoons canola oil
- 1/2 cup additional all-purpose flour, or as much as needed
- 1 package of active dry yeast
- 1/3 cup white sugar
- 2/3 cup warm water
- 2 cups all-purpose flour
- 1 cup bread flour, any brand

Directions:

1. In a bowl, dissolve the sugar and yeast in the water and let stand for 10 minutes.

2. In a large bowl, mix 2 cups all-purpose flour, the bread flour, corn oil and kosher salt; add the yeast mixture and stir until well combined.
3. Use the 1/2 cup of additional flour and dust a level work surface. Pour the dough onto the surface and knead the dough until smooth.
4. Oil a clean bowl and let the dough rise in it for 2 hours or until it doubles in size.
5. Place the dough on a pizza pan and top as desired.

Basic Pizza Sauce

Ingredients:

- 1 teaspoon oregano, dried
- Salt and pepper to taste
- 1/2 teaspoon sugar (optional)
- 2 tablespoons olive oil
- 1 can (28 ounces) whole tomatoes, crushed and undrained
- 1 onion, finely diced
- 1 minced clove of garlic
- 4 fresh leaves of basil

Directions:

1. In a heavy saucepan, cook the onions and garlic in the olive oil for 2 minutes.
2. Add the tomatoes; season with salt and pepper. Bring the mixture to a simmer and

add the basil and oregano, as well as the sugar if using.

3. Reduce the heat to slow simmer, cover and cook for 20 minutes or until thickened. Season again as needed.
4. Cool the sauce down and store (covered) in the refrigerator for up to 1 week if not using immediately.

Heirloom Pizza Sauce

Ingredients:

- 2 tablespoons parmesan cheese, grated
- 1 teaspoon each: dried oregano and basil
- 1/2 teaspoon each: salt and sugar
- 1/4 teaspoon pepper
- 1 bay leaf
- 1 teaspoon fennel seed
- 1 tablespoon butter
- 2 tablespoons olive oil
- 1/2 cup chopped onion
- 1/4 cup chopped celery
- 1 minced clove of garlic
- 1 can (8 ounces) tomato sauce
- 1 can (6 ounces) tomato paste

Directions:

1. In a skillet, sauté the onion, celery and garlic in a mixture of the oil and butter for 5 minutes or until transparent.
2. Add the tomato sauce and paste; stir until smooth.
3. Add the remaining Ingredients:.
4. Bring the mixture to a slow simmer and cook for 60 minutes, or until done to your taste.
5. Remove the bay leaf before using or storing.

Pizza Tentazione

Ingredients:

Dough:

- 2 tbsp. l. olive oil
- 1 tsp salt
- 5 g of dry yeast
- 2 cups of flour
- 1 cup warm water

Sauce:

- Basil to taste
- Oregano to taste
- Salt to taste
- 1 cup tomato juice
- 1 tomato
- 1 clove of garlic
- 3 tbsp. olive oil

- Ground black pepper to taste

Filling:

- 200 g of hard cheese
- Fresh parsley to taste
- Salt to taste
- 1 tbsp. vegetable oil for greasing the pan
- 150 g mushrooms
- 150 g of sausages
- 2 medium tomatoes

Directions:

Test preparation:

1. On the table Sift 2 cups flour. On top of the hill make a hole in and pour 2 cups of warm water, 2 tbsp. olive oil, add 1 tsp 5 g of salt and dry yeast.
2. Gently mix and start kneading the dough.
3. Knead the dough should be for 10 minutes, until it becomes elastic.

4. Large bowl sprinkle the flour and place the dough in it.
5. Cover with a damp towel and put in a warm dry place for 1 hour.

Sauce preparation:
1. Heat the pan, pour 3 tbsp. olive oil. Add finely chopped clove of garlic and fry until golden brown. Pour 1 cup of tomato juice and fry for 5 minutes. Add the chopped tomato and spices: basil, oregano, salt and pepper. Fry for another 5 minutes, stirring occasionally. Remove from heat and let cool. Cooked sauce through a sieve.

Preparation of the filling:
2. Finely chop all the Ingredients: and cheese grate.
3. After the dough has come, it needs to mash and roll out to a thickness of 0.5-1 cm.
4. Grease the pan with vegetable oil and put the dough.

5. Then the dough to grease prepared sauce and put the stuffing: sausage, mushrooms, tomatoes, parsley and cheese. Season with salt.
6. Bake 10-15 minutes in the preheated oven to 230 C. Bon appetite!

Pizza Dough With Cheese

Ingredients:

- 1 tsp soda
- 2 eggs
- 1 tbsp. Sahara
- 4 tbsp. sour cream
- 2 cups of flour
- 250 g of cottage cheese
- 100 g butter (melted)
- 1 tsp salt

Directions:

1. Cottage cheese mix well with eggs Masher. Lightly season with salt.
2. Soda mixed with sour cream and set aside.
3. Melt butter, cool slightly and pour into the cheese. Add the sour cream with sugar and baking soda. Mix well.

4. Pour the flour little by little, mix all until smooth.
5. Roll out the dough through the plastic wrap that is not torn, lay on a baking sheet and add any toppings for pizza and sprinkle with cheese.
6. Oven at 180 degrees for 30-35 minutes.

Pizza Roasted Garlic Lasagna Pizza

Ingredients:

- 2 tablespoons tomato paste
- 2 cups milk
- 2 tablespoons butter
- 2 tablespoons flour
- 2 cups shredded provolone cheese
- ½ cup parmesan cheese, grated, plus more for serving
- ½ pound pizza dough, store-bought or homemade
- 1 cup mozzarella cheese, shredded
- Chopped parsley, for garnish
- 1 head garlic
- 4 ounces pancetta, chopped (optional)
- 3 tablespoons olive oil

- 1 red pepper, diced
- ½ pound ground spicy Italian chicken sausage or ground chicken
- Kosher salt + pepper
- 1 (28 ounce) can crushed tomatoes

Directions:

1. To roast the garlic, preheat the oven to 400 degrees F. Chop off the top portion of the garlic head to reveal cloves. Peel any excess paper/skin off from the bulb of garlic. Place the cloves in a garlic roaster and drizzle with a teaspoon of olive oil. Cover and transfer to the oven and roast for 45 minutes, or until the garlic is golden brown and soft. Remove from the oven and allow to cool five minutes. Squeeze the garlic out of the paper skin into a bowl and mash well with a fork.

2. Position your pizza stone on the upper 1/3 rack of your oven. Preheat your oven to 500 degrees F. or as high as it can possibly go.
3. In a heavy bottomed pot, cook 1 tablespoon of olive oil and the pancetta over high heat, stirring, until the pancetta is lightly browned, about 3 minutes. Add 1 tablespoon of olive oil to the center of the pan and crumble in the ground sausage. Cook without stirring for 3 minutes, then begin breaking up the meat. Continue to cook, stirring occasionally, until well browned, about 5 minutes. Add the tomatoes, tomato paste, ½ cup milk, the roasted garlic, salt and pepper to the pot. Simmer the sauce, stirring occasionally until thickened, about 10-15 minutes. Taste to season with salt and pepper.
4. Meanwhile, melt the butter in a small saucepan over medium heat. Add the flour and cook, whisking constantly, for 1 minute.

Whisk in the remaining 1½ cups milk in a steady stream. Bring to a boil and cook for 2 minutes, whisking consistently. Remove from the heat, stir in the provolone cheese and then add the Parmesan. Season with salt and pepper.

5. On a lightly floured surface, push/roll the dough out until it is very thin.
6. Transfer the dough to a parchment paper lined baking sheet.
7. Spread the white sauce over the dough and then spread evenly with the meat sauce.
8. Top with mozzarella and evenly place the pepperoni over the cheese.
9. Carefully slide the pizza onto the hot stone and bake for 10-12 minutes or until the cheese is melted and bubbly.
10. Remove from the oven, garnish with parsley and Parmesan and serve.

Pizza Blt Ranch Flatbread Pizza

Ingredients:

- Shredded lettuce (I used about 1-2 lettuce leaves)
- Quartered grape tomatoes (I used 4-5 tomatoes per flatbread)
- Crumbled bacon (I used about 3-4 slices of cooked bacon per flatbread)
- Pre-made flatbreads
- Ranch dressing to taste (I used 1 tables spoon per flatbread but it depends on the size of the flatbread)

Directions:

1. Preheat the oven to 400 degrees and line a pan with parchment or foil (for easy clean up).
2. Place the flatbreads onto the pan and bake for 10-15 minutes until the edges brown slightly.
3. Remove and cool for a few minutes.

4. Spread ranch dressing onto each flat bread in a thin layer.
5. Top with lettuce tomatoes and bacon to taste.
6. Slice and enjoy!

Fast On Bread Pizza

Ingredients:

- 3 cloves of minced garlic
- 2 tomatoes
- 100 g of cheese
- 12-15 slices of salami
- 2 pickles
- 1 bar or flat bread loaf
- 3 tbsp. mayonnaise
- 3 tbsp. ketchup

Directions:
1. Bread cut in half lengthwise.
2. Mix ketchup and mayonnaise, add passed through a press garlic, mix well. The resulting sauce to grease bread.

3. Put the finely chopped tomatoes, then salami and sliced cucumbers. Sprinkle with cheese. Bake in the oven until golden brown.

Pizza With Salami And Tomato

Ingredients:

- 100 g of salami sausages
- 1/2 onion
- 1 tomato
- 450 g pizza dough
- 50 g of vegetable salsa
- 150 g of cheese

Directions:
1. Pre-knead pizza dough according to any recipe or use a proven recipe. Roll out the dough into a round cake.
2. Coat tomato salsa or ketchup.
3. Sprinkle half of the cheese pizza.
4. Sausages cut into slices and spread over the dough.
5. Onions finely chop and sprinkle them a pizza.

6. Tomatoes cut into small pieces and put it on a pizza.
7. Sprinkle all the cheese.
8. Put the pan with the pizza in a preheated 200-degree oven. Bake until tender, 25-30 minutes.
9. The finished pizza cut into pieces and serve.

Pizza Turkey Pizza

Ingredients:

- ¼ cup parmesan cheese , shredded
- seasonings , basil, oregano, garlic or rosemary, salt and pepper
- toppings of choice , onions, tomatoes, kalamata olives, and basil
- 2 pound turkey , ground
- 2 eggs
- 1 cup low carb pizza sauce
- 2 cups mozzarella cheese , shredded

Directions:

1. Preheat oven to 450 degrees
2. Lay a piece of parchment paper onto, or grease a rimmed baking sheet (must have a lip).

3. In medium bowl, mix the meat, eggs, parmesan and spices (if using) with your hands until everything is well combined.
4. Press the meat into a circular shape on your baking sheet. I used a second piece of parchment paper on top and a rolling pin to flatten it out.
5. Cook until the turkey has cooked all the way through and no red is left – this took me about 25 minutes, but it depends on how thick you made your crust.
6. Once cooked through, remove from the oven and crank it up to broil.
7. Spread pizza sauce over meat, the mozzarella, and any toppings you'd like.
8. Return to the over and broil.
9. Watch closely, you only want to melt/brown the cheese, but at this temp the pizza can burn easily!

10. Allow the pizza to cook before cutting and enjoy!

Captain America Pizza

Ingredients:

- 1 cup pizza sauce pizza sauce
- 4 flour tortillas large flour tortillas
- 3 cups shredded mozzarella
- 2 cups pepperoni pepperoni
- 2 slices mozzarella
- 1 cup olives chopped black olives

Directions:

1. Pre-specified the oven to 350° and collected a huge cooking sheet along with parchment paper.
2. Working on the cooking food sheet, spread a covering of pizzas spices onto two tortillas

then top every with a slim layer of disposed mozzarella and pepperoni.
3. Place the leftover 2 tortillas on best.
4. Spread another coating of pizzas spices onto each quesadilla then cover each completely with mozzarella.
5. Make a huge ring of pepperoni, overlapping the slices, around the quesadilla, then make a smaller ring of pepperoni inside.
6. Making use of a star biscuit cutter, arrange dark olives in a star shape. Cook for 15 minutes, or until parmesan cheese is melted.

Carne Asada Pizza Recipe

Ingredients:

- 1 tablespoon cornmeal
- 1 ounce part-skim mozzarella cheese , shredded (about 1/4 cup)
- 1 ounce cheddar cheese , shredded (about 1/4 cup)
- 1 ounce queso fresco, crumbled (about 1/4 cup)
- 1 cup chopped seeded tomato
- 2 tablespoons fresh lime juice
- 2 tablespoons minced red onion
- sprig cilantro (optional)
- 12 ounces refrigerated fresh pizza dough
- 2 small poblano peppers
- 8 ounces flank steak, trimmed

- 1/2 teaspoon ground cumin
- 1/2 teaspoon chipotle chile powder
- 1/8 teaspoon salt
- cooking spray
- 1 small red onion , cut into 1/2-inch-thick rings
- 1/2 cup lower-sodium marinara sauce
- 1 tablespoon adobo sauce from 1 can chipotle chiles in adobo sauce

Directions:
1. Remove dough coming from refrigerator. Let endure at room temp, covered, for thirty minutes.
2. Preheat broiler to high.
3. Arrange poblanos over a foil-lined baking linen.
4. Broil 8 mins or until charred on all attributes, turning occasionally.

5. Place peppers in evade; close tightly. Permit stand quarter-hour. Remove and seed potatoes; discard skin, membrane whitening strips.
6. Step 4Place a new pizza stone or perhaps heavy sheet pan inside oven. Preheat cooker to 500° (keep pizza stone or perhaps baking sheet inside oven as that preheats).
7. Sprinkle steak with cumin, chipotle powder, in addition to salt. Heat a new grill pan above high temperature. Coat baking pan with cooking aerosol. Add steak to be able to pan; cook some minutes on each and every side or right up until well marked. Permit stand 5 minutes. Very finely slice steak throughout the grain.
8. Add onion bands to pan; barbeque grill 4 minutes on each of your side or till well marked. Put in place a bowl; protect with

plastic cover. Combine marinara plus adobo sauce.

9. Roll dough right into a 15 x 9-inch rectangle on the lightly floured surface area. Pierce dough liberally having a fork. Spread cornmeal on pizzas stone.
10. Place money on hot rock; bake at 500° for 5 moments.
11. Remove stone through oven. Spread spices mixture over money, leaving a 1/2-inch border; top equally with mozzarella plus cheddar.
12. Arrange poblano and onion slices over pizza; best with steak.
13. Sprinkle with queso fresco. Come back stone to stove; bake pizza nine minutes or till crust is carried out.
14. Mix tomato, juice, plus minced red onion; sprinkle tomato combination over pizza.
15. Best with cilantro sprigs, if desired.

Cauliflower Breakfast Pizza

Ingredients:

- 1 teaspoon paprika
- kosher salt
- freshly ground black pepper
- 1 tablespoon extra-virgin olive oil
- 1 large onion
- 2 red bell peppers, chopped
- 1 cup ham
- 1 1/2 cups . shredded monterey jack
- 1 large head cauliflower
- 8 large eggs , divided
- 1 cup shredded white cheddar
- 2 cloves garlic , minced
- freshly chopped chives , for garnish

Directions:

1. Preheat oven to 425º and line the baking sheet along with parchment.
2. Grate cauliflower on small part of box grater to form fine crumbs. Transfer to a big bowl.
3. To dish add 2 ovum, white cheddar, garlic clove, and paprika plus season with salt and pepper. Mix until combined.
4. Move dough to ready baking sheet and dab right into a crust.
5. Cook until golden plus dried up, 25 moments.
6. Meanwhile, inside a sizable skillet above moderate heat, temperature essential oil.
7. Put onion plus potatoes and prepare right up until soft, eight mins.
8. Stir within pork. Within a little pan, whisk with the other remaining 6 ovum and season alongside with salt in addition to spice up.

9. Fill eggs in to be able to skillet and scramble, 4 minutes.
10. Get rid of cauliflower crust coming from stove and temperature broiler.
11. Spread a new slim layer regarding salsa on leading.
12. Best with screwed up ovum and Monterey jack port.
13. Pan until parmesan mozzarella cheese is golden, a couple of minutes. Garnish alongside with chives and performance.

Individual Pizza Doughs

Ingredients:

- 1/2 teaspoon salt
- 2 tablespoons olive oil
- Extra flour for kneading and extra oil for the bowl
- 1/2 cup warm water
- 1/2 teaspoon sugar
- 1 1/2 teaspoons yeast, dry
- 1 1/2 cups all-purpose flour, or bread flour

Directions:

1. Mix the water, yeast and sugar together in a bowl; set aside for 15 minutes until foamy.
2. Combine the flour and salt in a large bowl and mix well.
3. Make a well in the center and add the olive oil along with the yeast mixture.

4. Stir the contents with a fork until it forms a dough; pour it onto a floured surface.
5. With hands, knead the dough for about 5 minutes or until smooth.
6. Oil a large bowl with olive oil; put the dough into the bowl and turn several times to coat with oil.
7. This will keep the top of the dough from drying out while it rises. Let the dough rise for 1 hour or until it has doubled in size.
8. When it has risen, use a dough cutter or serrated knife to cut the dough into six portions and shape into small pizzas.
9. Top as desired and bake at 475 degrees for about 15 minutes.

www.ingramcontent.com/pod-product-compliance
Lightning Source LLC
Chambersburg PA
CBHW050238120526
44590CB00016B/2135